Losing the woman within

By

Linda Parkinson-Hardman

Cover image © Photographer: Judy Ben Joud | Agency: Dreamstime.com
ISBN 13: 978-1-4303-0276-6

The Hysterectomy Association
www.hysterectomy-association.org.uk

Contents

This Book is dedicated to my parents, Pat and Alf.

Time cools, time clarifies; no mood can be maintained
quite unaltered through the course of hours.
Mark Twain

Welcome to Losing the woman within

A hysterectomy can, and does, relieve many women of symptoms that are distressing and that have a very profound effect on the quality of their life. It can literally be a life saver and will probably mean a new lease of life, not only for you, but for your family as well. Depending on the condition that has led you to this decision, your life will be completely different after having the operation. You won't have to worry about tampons and towels or pain and discomfort any more. However, the recovery process will involve not only your physical body, but your emotions as well and this book has been written to help you navigate your way to the new happy and healthy self you will be in months to come.

When I had my hysterectomy, I found myself lost in a sea of bewildering thoughts, feelings and practical necessities. I had imagined that as soon as the operation was over, I would be 'a new woman', just like the gynaecologist had told me and was extremely concerned, guilty, and angry – at myself - when I wasn't. As the years have gone by, I have come to realise that what I felt was perfectly normal, that there is no 'right way' to have a hysterectomy – there is only the way we each individually experience it and there are so many shades of experience they make a veritable rainbow of alternatives.

Since I started The Hysterectomy Association back in 1996, I have been in contact with many women over the years, and as I listened to their stories I became more convinced than ever, that one important key – *perhaps the most important one* - to our long term health is a simple acknowledgement of how our hysterectomy makes us feel. The title '*Losing the Woman Within*' is in response to the huge numbers of women that contact The Hysterectomy Association from all over the world every year fearing that a hysterectomy will profoundly affect their essential womanhood.

This book is one way of looking at the emotions surrounding a hysterectomy. I have used my own experiences (highlighted with a different typeface), and those of the 1000's of women who have been in touch with The Hysterectomy Association, to illustrate the sorts of things I am talking about. There is also the opportunity to use it as a personal journal, for you to record your own journey to wellness. You can use the journal as much, or as little, as you want; its purpose is to help you navigate your own operation and recovery. It is entirely up to you – but I would strongly recommend that if you are going through some emotional turmoil following your hysterectomy, that you acknowledge your feelings. Talking is good, but if you can't find someone to talk to, then writing or drawing can be very cathartic. I have also included a few activities that I have found effective in my counselling practice, but they are only a guide, you may have a different way of considering your situation.

Introduction

It would be true to say that most women will experience some kind of emotional upheaval after a hysterectomy, but the depth of emotion will be very personal to each and every one. There is no 'right' or 'wrong' way to experience a hysterectomy – there is only your own unique way of doing so, which will depend on a huge number of different factors, some of which you may never have any control over. Having said that, this book is not meant to be predictive in any shape or form it is really all about giving you permission to experience the emotions you have without feeling that you *should be doing, or feeling something different'.*

I had my own hysterectomy when I was 32 years old as a result of gynaecological problems I had had since I was about 16. I had my womb, ovaries, fallopian tubes, cervix and the top portion of my vagina removed. I didn't know then, what I know now – but boy do I wish I had; I may have had an easier time emotionally than I did and I may have stopped being so hard on myself for being weak, as I thought. I expected to be back at work within six weeks and I assumed that I would feel fine as soon as the physical pain had stopped.

How wrong I was. I ended up being off work for several months and my emotions were on a roller coaster – one day I was up and the next I was down – and I couldn't work out why it all seemed so difficult. This wasn't how my gynaecologist had painted the picture for me; I was supposed to be a 'new woman' within six weeks. I blamed myself for my lack of backbone and strength of character; what was worse though was that I allowed others to also blame my weak will as well, which just made me feel . even worse. I recovered physically very well eventually – but my feelings were rent apart.

But, here I am eleven years later and I have a new life, better health than I have ever experienced before and a renewed sense of purpose. I even have a new husband as well. It didn't take me eleven years to get to this point though (I wouldn't want to worry you). My real recovery started when I finally began to give a voice to my feelings and if there was one thing I could wish for everyone reading this book, it would be the gift of giving you permission to feel any way you do, at any given time and at any point before, during or after your hysterectomy.

So just what sorts of things *might* you experience? Well, they could be grouped into two distinct types of reaction; physical, and emotional. They may include things like anxiety, stress, guilt, grief, depression, or even post traumatic stress. As I said, most of us will experience some of these, to a greater or lesser degree, and you may experience them for a wide variety of reasons, hormonal, menopausal or even psychological, but the important thing to remember is that they are not 'wrong'. They are your own unique expression of what having a hysterectomy means to you, the wonderful, thoughtful, kind, loving, beautiful person that is reading this book.

Physical Effects of Hysterectomy

There are many physical effects to a hysterectomy; some are more obvious than others such as post operative discomfort, bleeding for a short while, difficulty doing anything physical for several weeks or even months, tiredness, exhaustion and insomnia.

It is important to remember that your physical response to a hysterectomy will be as individual as your emotional response. There is no 'right' or 'wrong' way to recover; there is just recovery, and it could be easy for you to become disheartened if you don't feel you are recovering as quickly as the agenda given you by the gynaecologist says you will. When you feel like this, it is incredibly important that you 'go with the flow' of what **your** own needs are, not those of some fictional perfect patient. Remember that the 'average patient' is based on a range of women aged between 20 – 80, who all have a wide variety of symptoms and problems, will have had very different operations and who had vastly different social and support experiences. In these circumstances, there can be no 'average' – as there is no average woman.

All sorts of factors can help, or hinder, your physical recovery – and you won't be able to control all of them. They are things like what your health was like before your operation; how fit you are; your age; whether you have a good system of support at home so you can relax and take things easy; the sort of job you do;

whether you have responsibilities you can't pass to anyone else (such as young children or caring for a relative) and whether there is anyone you can talk to about how you feel. All of these things play an important role in your physical and emotional well being. So, try not to be hard on yourself – you can only get well as quickly as you are able to and tales of your friends' Aunty Flo, who was up and about doing the laundry a week after her hysterectomy, should be taken with a very, very, large pinch of salt *(but no more than 6gms a day mind!).*

You may also have the slightly surreal feeling that something is missing from your body and it has been described in various ways by different women, but could be felt as:

- ❖ a change in the way your abdomen feels
- ❖ a hollow or space in your tummy
- ❖ the muscles and other organs shifting around inside
- ❖ a pulling, or dragging sensation especially when you lie on one side (a pillow under your tummy can really help with this one).

Not everyone is this aware of their body though, and many of you may not even notice that there is any change at all to the way your body feels physically.

Menopause Mayhem

The menopause is a natural part of the ageing process and it is caused by the changes in the levels of female sex hormones in your body as you get older. The hormones that precipitate most of the menopausal symptoms are falling levels of oestrogen and progesterone. Normally, we would go on producing small amounts of these hormones, as well as testosterone, well past our fifties, and our menopause would be gradual. We would also normally continue to produce testosterone for up to 20 years after menopause.

The menopause is a little like going through puberty in reverse, so any mood swings that you have as a result of the menopause, may well exacerbate any emotional turmoil you are already feeling. In some cases, the menopause could be the sole reason for your difficult feelings so forewarned is forearmed, as they say.

If you haven't yet gone through the menopause and you have your ovaries removed then you will go through the menopause immediately. There is no escaping this, it will happen. Your body will experience a sudden drop in hormone levels, and depending on your age, this could be traumatic. As a result of this you may experience any, or all, of the most common menopausal symptoms.

When we have a surgical menopause then the change in hormone levels is swift and dramatic. Not only do we lose most of our oestrogen and progesterone, but we also lose our testosterone as well. The effect on our emotions of this hormonal loss can be quite devastating. The hormonal impact on an already emotionally charged situation can tip you over the edge, especially if you aren't getting enough rest.

I have never talked to a woman who has experienced all of the symptoms you can have with the menopause - but everyone has a few, and the ones they do have seem to change over time as well. It might be helpful to tick each of those symptoms you are experiencing in the list below, because then you can talk to your GP about what your options are, after eliminating any other possible causes for them of course.

Symptom	Tick	Symptom	Tick
Hot flushes (flashes)	❏	Night Sweats	❏
Headaches	❏	Insomnia	❏
Palpitations or irregular heart beat	❏	Mood swings	❏
Dry vagina, which can cause pain when you have sex	❏	Tiredness (over and above normal post surgical tiredness)	❏
Difficulty concentrating	❏	Memory lapses	❏
Itchy skin – could feel like crawling	❏	Urinary incontinence	❏
Breast tenderness	❏	Aching muscles, joints and tendons	❏
Muscle tension	❏	Gastrointestinal upsets, such as diarrhoea, wind, bloating, flatulence	❏
Depression	❏	Increase in allergies	❏
Weight gain	❏	Thinning hair	❏
Feeling light headed or dizziness	❏	Change in body odour	❏
Tingling in the arms and legs	❏	Increase in bleeding gums	❏
Burning sensation in the mouth	❏	Changes in fingernails	❏
Changes in skin texture and tone	❏	Loss of interest in sex	❏
Tinnitus (ringing in the ears)	❏	Feelings of unspecific fear and dread	❏
Increased facial hair growth	❏	Severe anxiety/panic attacks	❏
Breasts may shrink slightly	❏	Vaginal walls thinning and susceptible to infection	❏

For those of you who did not have your ovaries removed, it would be helpful to be aware of this list of possible symptoms because research has shown that 50% of you are likely to experience ovarian failure within five years of your hysterectomy, and most of you will probably go through menopause a couple of years earlier than you might otherwise have done. The reasons for this aren't really clear, but it could have something to do with the blood supply to the ovaries being disrupted by the surgery. A good indicator, by the way, of when you might have expected to have your menopause naturally, would be when your mother started hers, as there does seem to be a strong genetic link.

If you think you are starting to have menopausal symptoms, then a blood oestrogen test from your doctor would be recommended; they aren't completely accurate, but can be helpful in giving an indication of the start of menopause. If you would prefer not to have a blood test, you can also buy urine tests as well.

When I had my hysterectomy, I had my ovaries removed. I was 32 years old and my menopausal symptoms started within 24 hours of surgery. I was immediately put on hormone patches and although my physical symptoms – hot flushes and night sweats – were alleviated, this actually triggered a return of the endometriosis, *which was precisely the reason I had my hysterectomy in the first place!*

So, several months down the line, I was advised to stop using HRT for up to 12 months to allow all the cysts to die back completely. I experienced very severe menopausal symptoms – the worst happened to be the night sweats, which gave me insomnia and added to my emotional overload. I hate to say it, but I became very bitter and twisted. I particularly resented anyone telling me how good a night's sleep they had had – especially my husband, whose duty (I felt) was to be by my side, going through the same hell I was enduring. I actually remember prodding him in the back every time he fell asleep to make sure he stayed awake with me!

However, I did become a little more considerate when he gently pointed out that he actually had to get some sleep so that he could go to work to earn a crust so we could eat the next day.

I have now been back on HRT for about 10 years and haven't had a problem since. I will probably continue to take it until I would naturally have gone through the menopause - age 50ish - and then will think about doing something more 'natural' to maintain my health.

Emotional Reactions to Hysterectomy

The reasons for our emotional reactions to a hysterectomy can be many and varied. For instance, our hormones finely tune the balance in our bodies systems; when we go through the menopause - either surgically or naturally - this hormonal balance is upset. Our hormones also help to regulate how we feel by creating our 'happy feelings'. This means that sometimes it can be difficult to tell - especially for those of us who had our ovaries removed - whether what we feel is due to hormonal deficiency, and would therefore benefit from supplementing with hormones, or whether there is more deep seated cause that is possibly psychological.

Anxiety and Stress

One of the most common emotional responses to a hysterectomy usually occurs before the operation ever takes place. The anxiety and stress levels that most women experience will go through the roof as they try to manage their way through it. They often put their own fears on the back burner as they try to put in place all the mechanisms to manage the home and family for the period that they will be in hospital and/or recuperating.

I could go so far as to say every woman will have some degree of anxiety about the operation and about how well they will cope with it. I would also venture the assumption that all women create huge amounts of stress for themselves as they make sure that there is enough food in the freezer, the shopping has been done, the house has been cleaned and the dog will be walked twice a day!

But, it is vital that you also give yourself the time and space to look at your own anxieties about the operation. Reducing your stress levels is one way of ensuring that you will recover as quickly as possible. This is because stress increases a variety of hormones in the body, which prevent our immune system from working as well as it could.

My own anxieties were mainly about dying on the operating table. I coped with them by ignoring them, and spent the month before the operation buying Christmas presents, wrapping them, writing cards and sending them, cooking Christmas dinner and putting it in the freezer and cleaning every single nook and cranny I could find. (I actually had my operation on 4th November, so I think I was a little hasty doing all this at the beginning of October – but I guess it takes all sorts!).

I also felt guilty about abandoning my employer for six weeks, and worked longer hours to make sure everything was absolutely up to date, wrote copious notes for colleagues who would be covering my absence and generally made myself ill. I've later learnt to acknowledge that, no matter what my various employers have said over the years, they always coped without me – and the reams of instructions I always left were usually unread.

After the operation I found that I was crying over all the things that could have gone wrong while I was in hospital, I could have died, a knife could have slipped, and I could have picked up a major infection. I didn't manage to connect them to my fear of dying on the operating table though. Later on, when I was training to be a counsellor, I realised I felt I had literally 'put my life on the line' when I had my hysterectomy; and that the stress of this, coupled with the fact that I had been too afraid to ask the question "will I die" actually increased the levels of stress hormones in my body and so prevented my body (and my emotions) from healing as quickly as they would otherwise have done.

I am going to suggest that you draw up a list of your own anxieties about having a hysterectomy. Be as honest with yourself as you can be right now – you can always come back to it later if you wish. Then, when you have a list of your fears, talk to the people you think can help you to put them into perspective. They might include your gynaecologist, or anaesthetist, your husband, your family, your GP or maybe best of all, your closest friends. However, don't forget that you can ask your questions and share your experiences with the other women that use our forums.
(www.hysterectomy-association.org.uk/forums).

Acknowledging Our Fears – why not think about completing one of these simple forms for each fear you have; you can photocopy extra forms at the back of the book as required. Describe your fear as fully as you can, be descriptive, actually have an image in your mind when you do this exercise and really feel the fear as you write. When you have a very clear idea of what your fear is, you can then decide who you need to talk to. It can be helpful to write down the sorts of things you want to ask or things your want to say so that you can practice beforehand if necessary.

Make as many notes as you can, and if you are talking to your doctor or gynaecologist you might find it helps to take a friend or your partner along as they may hear things that were said that you missed for some reason.

Take as long as you want to do this exercise and you might want to deal with just one thing at a time, perhaps working up to your greatest fear when you have some experience of things improving. It might also be helpful to read right through this book first, and come back to this activity later on. This is because some of your fears might be helped by the information you are reading.

MY FEAR IS?

I WILL TALK TO THE FOLLOWING PEOPLE ABOUT IT

THEIR ANSWER WAS ....

Once you have completed this exercise, you will probably find that, although you still have some fear, it is less than it was. This is because the fear of something happening is often more frightening and difficult cope with than the reality. Fear is an emotion that effectively 'freezes' the logical processing part of our brain – a bit like being a rabbit caught in a car' headlight.

After a hysterectomy, your anxiety and stress levels could still be extremely high. This can happen for any number of reasons such as the incredible tiredness you will feel and the irritation that this brings as you find yourself unable to cope with even simple things that weren't a problem before your operation. It could be caused by the trauma many people have following any form of major surgery. And it may also be due to the high levels of stress hormones that our bodies produce in anticipation of putting ourselves 'at risk' by submitting our bodies to a surgeons knife. The key to dealing with this sort of stress and anxiety is to practice relaxation techniques and by giving yourself the time and space to recover at your own pace.

Reducing Stress Levels

There are a variety of things you can do to help reduce your stress levels in the run up to a hysterectomy, and they are also suitable for helping you to relax after the operation as well. One of the simplest is to do the following gentle breathing exercise while listening to soothing instrumental music. If you don't have anything suitable we have a number of CD's which you can buy with guided relaxation exercises on them. You can find them by visiting our online store at:

http://www.hysterectomy-association.org.uk/shop/catalog.php

Find yourself somewhere comfortable and quiet to sit or lie for 15 minutes or so where you won't be disturbed by visitors or telephones. Put the music on and settle yourself down. Close your eyes and concentrate on your breathing. Just pay attention to your breath going in and out. Don't try to analyse it or correct it in any way, just notice how it goes. If you become aware of your mind wandering, gently bring it back to being aware of your breathing. Don't worry if you fall asleep, as this is a good indicator that you need the extra rest. Stay like this for at least 15 minutes everyday – and slowly your stress levels will reduce, you'll feel calmer and more peaceful in your normal day to day activities.

Anger

Many women I talk to report that they feel very angry before and after a hysterectomy. When this is coupled with other emotions as well, it can be very draining on our energy levels. The key to dealing with anger is working out why you are angry in the first place. Is it at your body for letting you down like this, or perhaps it might be at your husband or partner for being over protective or not supportive enough, or perhaps it could be at the medical profession for not spotting your problem earlier or forcing you into this surgery without giving you any alternatives. Whatever the reason – logical or not, accept that you feel angry and that you have a right to feel angry – it is perfectly normal and natural to feel this way at such a time. Acknowledge your anger and who it is directed against and once you have done this, you will then be in a position to deal with it.

Recipe for dealing with anger
Ingredients:
One Pillow
One large Bed
Two hands
Take the pillow, put it on your bed, make your hands into fist and then bash the pillow. As you do this, you may feel very silly at first, but as you get into it – it becomes easier, and you

may find that a lot of pent up emotions begin to be released.
You might find yourself crying, shouting or even screaming.
Whatever happens – do it until you don't feel you need to do it
anymore, you can always do it again tomorrow if you need to.
If you are at all shy about expressing your emotions, you might
find it easier to do when all the family are out

Grief

It is true to say that almost everyone who has a hysterectomy
will experience some degree of grief. Whether this is simply the
post-operative blues - which is common with many surgical
procedures – or something more profound, will be entirely
dependent on the feelings each one of us has about ourselves as
women. It may also be related to the levels of stress hormones
that our bodies produce in order to manage the 'fight or flight'
response that, literally putting our lives on line by having
surgery, causes.

The post operative blues are often due to a chemical reaction in
the body that occurs for a wide variety of reasons, for instance:

- ❖ Anaesthetic can have this effect on the body, especially as
  it begins to be flushed out of the system
- ❖ Pain, tiredness, weakness and dizziness will all contribute
  as well; and having too many people with unrealistic
  expectations of your recovery can be quite draining
- ❖ You may have been so excited about having a
  hysterectomy that will finally relieve all the troublesome
  problems you have been living with that you create a sort

of euphoria about it. This will encourage the body to produce excess chemical substances like steroids, adrenaline, or endorphins. After your operation, these chemicals stop being produced which can produce a sort of withdrawal effect.

Most of these are usually short lived, and will end when your normal hormone balance begins to reassert itself.

> Tip. One way of dealing with some of the post operative blues is to drink plenty of water as this helps to flush toxins like the anaesthetic out of your body. Another good idea is to walk as pumping the muscles in this way has a similar flushing effect.

A more deep-seated grief however, is something entirely different from these transitory feelings and is usually related to how we see ourselves as women. For many women having a hysterectomy cuts to the very heart of what being a woman is all about. We have wombs, we are the mothers of our species, we bear children and nurture them until they are old enough to make their own way and even then we worry about them not wearing their vests. You may feel it because you never had the chance to have children, because you can't have any more children or because a part of you that was the 'essence of your womanhood' has been taken away from you. It is essentially associated with how we deal with any change in life and can be summarised as a change of circumstance of any type that produces a loss of some kind.

The intensity of your grief is going to be related to how your loss is perceived. If you feel that it is not significant, then your grief will be minimal or barely felt. But there may also be a whole range of emotions that you experience with your loss – whatever it is you feel you have lost; your womb, dreams, choice about your body and future, or the hope of having children.

One way of dealing with all of these emotions is to do 'grief work'. The acronym TEAR explains it very well:

T = taking in, and accepting, the reality of the loss (womb, hope, dream, longed for child)

E = experiencing the pain of the loss

A = adjusting to the new environment that no longer has the lost 'thing' in it

R = reinvesting in the new reality

What this sort of work requires you to do is to allow yourself the time, space and opportunity to experience all the feelings you have about your operation. Try writing down how you feel about the whole experience and about what you have lost and why. You could write it in the form of a letter to yourself, the womb you have lost or the child you may never have. Either way, whatever you feel should be allowed to come out. There may be lots of tears and/or anger – but no-one need see what you are writing except you.

All sorts of things can set you off and it can be helpful - at least initially - to have a stack of weepy films to hand, because you can then release some of your feelings without having to explain to everyone why you feel the way you do every five minutes. Thoughts about not having children, never getting better, no longer being a woman, never having another period and 'being different now' should be acknowledged and accepted as a part of your recovery. Don't suppress them - it is vitally important that you acknowledge your feelings and emotions otherwise they could become like a snowball that rolls down a hill, getting bigger and bigger.

Of all the emotional issues that are often raised after having a hysterectomy, never having a child can be the most heart rending of all. Some of us who are in this situation will experience this as a huge sense of loss because bearing children may have been a large part of our life expectations. As a result we may begin to question what it was all about. We may feel angry at our bodies for having let us down, or at ourselves for not being stronger, and it can take a long time to work through these emotions. We may also have to deal with the unfulfilled expectations of many others around us, such as our partner, parents, relatives and even friends.

The sight of a woman with a new baby, or - as my mother often does to me - the 'phone call saying "did I know that such and such from school had just had another baby" can be triggers we react to instantly and immediately, pushing our buttons and leaving us angry, drained and sad all at the same time.

We may even have put off having children as well because of career demands or other life experiences we wanted first; these can trigger feelings of guilt, and we may now be feeling that we were stupid to wait, or that we had been too selfish somehow.

However, not everyone who didn't have children before a hysterectomy will be affected in such a dramatic way, particularly if they had never expected to have a family anyway. But sometimes it's not the decision that defines our reaction, but when the choice is taken away from us. Up until the point we have a hysterectomy, we still have a choice about whether or not to have children (in theory at least!), but once the operation removes that choice, then grief can also come as a shock to the career woman who had never expected it to concern her.

And lets not forget that even those who do have children are not immune from these feelings either; they can be just as intense regardless of whether you believed you had completed your family before hysterectomy.

Dealing with all of these emotions requires time and sensitivity, not only from those around you, but also from yourself. They are not going to be gone overnight and you may find that they linger for months, or when they are not dealt with at the time, even years after your surgery.

The most important step is to simply acknowledge your feelings first and then see if you can find the courage to talk about how you feel. Setting boundaries with well meaning friends and family about what you do, and don't want to talk about, can be very helpful in avoiding 'touchy' subjects, until you are in a better space to deal with them. And, if you find that you aren't able to talk to anyone close to you, then perhaps talking with a counsellor who specialises in women's issues or bereavement might be beneficial.

I had been unable to have children before I had my hysterectomy, and although I had always said I never wanted to have them anyway, and that losing my womb wouldn't be a problem; I was shocked to find how hard it was to cope with my emotions. It wasn't so much not being able to have children that mattered to me, it was the fact that I no longer had the option of 'changing my mind' if I wanted to. And my womb! I hadn't appreciated how much it was a part of me — it defined me as a woman, men didn't have them — so had I suddenly become less of a woman and more male?

I was very confused about how I felt; I oscillated between hope and despair, and much of the time I pretended everything was OK, even to myself. It took a long time to accept that it was alright to feel the way I did, and when I did achieve that I gained release from my own mental torment.

Depression

When you are depressed, you may hate yourself and feel frightened that other people will only see your negatives. You may cut yourself off from them, because you don't want to disappoint them. Every time you look at yourself, you find something else to blame – your past is full of how bad you have been and your future doesn't look much better. It can be a prison that you can find no way out of, and where love and compassion are not allowed to visit. It often occurs after some sort of loss, which could be recent – in the case of your operation – or it could be in the unexorcised memories and feelings from the distant past, which your hysterectomy brings back to you.

Clinical depression is usually caused by a chemical imbalance in the brain; these chemical imbalances can be caused by a variety of things such as illness, trauma and shock. You may suffer depression after a hysterectomy for any number of reasons, but the most likely cause is going to be unresolved grief about something. The symptoms of depression may include:

❖ feeling tired all the time and with diminished activity.
❖ losing interest in life or with an ability to enjoy yourself.
❖ reduced concentration and attention.
❖ reduced self-esteem/self-confidence.
❖ feelings of guilt and unworthiness.
❖ developing a bleak and pessimistic view of the future.
❖ thinking about or actually performing acts of self-harm/suicide.

❖ suffering disturbed sleep patterns, either early wakening, insomnia, the inability to get to sleep or get up in the morning and extreme lethargy.

❖ diminished appetite and self care.

If you have four or more symptoms from the list above, then it might be advisable to talk to your GP about how you are feeling. They may be able to help you with medication and/or counselling. For mild to moderate depression, you may find that herbal remedies such as St John's Wort are helpful (however, they may interact with other medication you are taking so I recommend asking your Pharmacist for advice).

Depression also prevents your immune system from functioning properly, and if you are still recovering from surgery then it may compromise the speed at which you return to full health.

Having said all that though, the prison of depression can, in a strange way, be a comforting place to be – it is a breathing space in your life that allows your mind and body to let go of old patterns of behaviour, thoughts and experiences. It has been described by Gwyneth Lewis in her book 'Sunbathing in the Rain', as "a very kind disorder" which "will only return if you refuse to learn the lessons it has to teach you". It can also heal itself without any intervention at all sometimes. In fact 30% of cases of depression do heal spontaneously, without either medication or counselling.

My grandmother died on Christmas day, 11 months before I had my hysterectomy. After her funeral, I had a breakdown – mainly because it had invoked memories of the death of my brother when I was 10 years old. I had never grieved for him and my grandmother's death brought everything back to me to be re-examined, and I found myself wanting. The thing that characterised my own depression was the inability to make a decision, if someone asked me what I wanted to eat, I would burst into tears; deciding what to wear was a nightmare and it was easier to stay in pj's and a dressing gown. Every time someone said 'it could be worse, think of the starving in Africa' it actually made it worse, because I then felt guilty for being depressed. I did take anti-depressants, and eventually returned to work part-time the following May. I also had counselling at the time, but I wasn't really ready for what it would expose of myself and it was only years later that I finally allowed myself to feel all the emotions I had buried in 1994.

I have always felt that my hysterectomy was, in some way, bound up in my depression – if I hadn't been depressed that year, would I have ended up having a hysterectomy? I will never know the answer to that fully – but at long last I am beginning to get a sense of what led me down the path to the operating table.

Post Traumatic Stress Disorder (PTSD)

PTSD is a phrase we often hear on news about victims and witnesses of a disaster; it may not be something we immediately recognise as being relevant in our own particular circumstances. Some recent research is beginning to suggest that it may be triggered by a hysterectomy. In fact, a hysterectomy can exhibit two of the characteristics that the American Psychiatric Association say must be experienced before a diagnosis of PTSD to be given – they are that "the person experienced an event that involved threatened death or serious injury" and that "the person's response involved fear, helplessness or horror".

There is incredible variance in the way in which people generally approach events such as a hysterectomy. Many will talk about what it was like to have a hysterectomy to anyone who will listen 'till the cows come home'. But others of us feel that it is a very private and personal experience and one that they would not want to share with anyone else. However, talking about your hysterectomy to another person, especially someone that has been there themselves, can be very therapeutic.

If you can't talk to someone either because there is no one to talk to, or because you feel inhibited in some way, then simply writing in a private journal can be helpful in acknowledging your feelings about your experience. If we are experiencing very strong feelings and we pretend to all and sundry, even ourselves, that there is nothing wrong and that everything is fine, we risk making things worse in the long run, because our emotions have a habit of tripping us up in the most unexpected of ways.

For instance, you may have had an argument with your husband or partner, which seemed to come out of the blue or may have been out of all proportion to the subject under discussion, but it later becomes obvious that you were feeling anxious about something else entirely. That is an incident where our emotions have tripped us up.

Guilt

Most women would say that they knew they might feel grief, anxiety and stress, but that they were completely unaware that they may also have a huge amount of guilt when they have a hysterectomy. What do I mean by guilt? Well, it's the feeling that you are somehow responsible for the situation that you find yourself in, and there are various reasons why it may rear its head. For instance:

❖ you may find that the relief you feel at ridding your body of the need to worry about periods and pain may suddenly seem a heavy price to pay for loss of child-bearing potential, even if you did not really want another child.

❖ there may have been expectations from your family to have children

❖ you may have decided to put off having children until you were settled in your career

❖ the degree of involvement you felt you had in the decision to have a hysterectomy may mean that you feel resentful

30

of what has been done *to you*, rather than feeling that you made the right decision for yourself.

❖ having children may have been a part of the 'marriage contract' with your husband

❖ or you may unconsciously be blaming yourself for decisions you made earlier in your life.

❖ you may have completed your family but feel guilty for those you met on your journey who couldn't have children

When I was 22 I became pregnant. It was completely out of the blue and unexpected; my reaction was to have the pregnancy terminated. As a result of the termination, I then suffered a severe pelvic infection which was made worse by endometriosis I already had. This left me with an inability to have children despite infertility treatment when I was in my late 20's. I told myself that it didn't matter because I had never really wanted children anyway. I hadn't realised how much anger I had at myself for my abortion until relatively recently – I now understand that I felt my endometriosis, the pelvic infection and my subsequent hysterectomy were a punishment that I had to suffer because I'd had the abortion. I felt a huge amount of guilt because I couldn't have children, because my parents would never be grandparents, and because my husband would make a fantastic father. Strangely though, I never wanted children for myself – it was all about fulfilling other people's expectations.

Your Relationship after Hysterectomy

Your most intimate relationships may be one of the areas of your life that has suffered the most over the years leading up to, and including, your hysterectomy. Your physical symptoms may have prevented you from getting involved in activities with your children, going out for the evening with your partner or even seriously compromised your sex life through pain, discomfort and bleeding.

Your hysterectomy may have been viewed by you and your family, as the answer to your prayers - a way of finally getting back to the woman you used to be. This could be somewhat unrealistic though, as you will have changed and grown older as the years have progressed and your relationships will have adapted over the years to account for your illness.

The vast majority of women do get through their hysterectomy well – they felt ready for it emotionally and physically, and it really does represent a new lease of life for them and their families.

For some of us however, our gynaecological problems may well have masked other, more fundamental problems in our relationships as it can be easy to put all the negative feelings we have down to the endometriosis, heavy bleeding or fibroids. With the hysterectomy, comes the expectation that everything will be 'alright now', and it can come as a shock to both of you if this expectation fails to materialise.

It would be true to say that we do get quite a lot of calls to our helpline from men, who are bewildered by changes in their partners' attitude to them, and a common comment is 'she doesn't want me any more'. It is difficult for them to understand why there is suddenly a change in your feelings. You may have known deep down – but been ignoring - for a long time that there was a problem, and you may believe it has been as obvious as the nose on your face that things weren't right; but if you have never voiced anything, it will come as a huge surprise to someone that isn't expecting it. It seems that our gynaecological problems may well overshadow other issues. When we have a hysterectomy that deals with our physical condition, it then forces these other issues into the spotlight where they can no longer be ignored.

We may also find ourselves looking to make changes in our lives because we no longer have to take account of the physical problems we had, and we now want to make up for the lost years. If this isn't matched by our partners' expectations, then there could be some conflict that will need to be resolved.

After a hysterectomy, it is important that you look at ways you can address the changes that may have occurred. This is probably easier with children as they are naturally more adaptable than adults - and will welcome a return to 'life' for their mum. Developing your constantly evolving relationship with your partner though, will be more complex and may take hours of talking and listening on both your parts.

Will I ever have sex again?

Generally your sex life should improve after hysterectomy. The conditions that you suffered from – pain, tiredness, feeling unwell all the time - are no longer there. You may have a greater sexual freedom particularly if you no longer have to worry about contraception, and the removal of your womb shouldn't affect the physical act of lovemaking. Researchers have also shown that most of us enjoy sex more as we get older anyway, probably because we no longer have the 'performance expectations' of our twenties and thirties, we are usually more at ease with our bodies and often have more time to enjoy it.

Many of us are nervous about our first sexual encounter after surgery, especially about experiencing pain, affecting any of the scars or even causing internal damage. In the majority of cases you will not have a problem physically, but the fear can be debilitating.

As far as the physical aspects of actual intercourse are concerned, it would be foolish to attempt to have sex before you have had the all clear. Your scar (if you have one) can be a good indicator of when all is healed; when it is the same colour as the rest of the skin around it, you will probably be healed inside as well. Any pink or redness means that there is still healing going on.

Having said that, although most women report their sex life improves, a small number may notice that there is something different about their sexual response and orgasm. This could be because a hysterectomy can cause some damage to the pelvic autonomic nerves, it may also disturb the blood flow to the pelvic region which could, in turn, have an effect on the way your body responds to normal sexual stimuli. A number of women have also reported that their experience of orgasm has changed and it is beginning to appear that the contraction and elevation of the womb during the arousal phase of sex and its subsequent pressure on the cervix, may play a significant part in the experience of orgasm for some of us - although many of us may never be aware of these physical responses at all.

Where you experience the most stimulation could also affect your sex life. If you are generally aroused to orgasm by clitoral stimulation, then the likelihood is that you won't experience any appreciable difference in your orgasm after your hysterectomy. If however, you are aroused by vaginal stimulation then you may experience some changes in the way in which orgasm feels.

If you are someone that is aware of the movements of your womb when you orgasm and you are at all concerned about your sex life, then it may be worth considering whether the payoff you get from having no bleeding, pain or discomfort after a hysterectomy is worth losing the intensity of your sexual experience for.

Physical changes after the menopause (either natural or surgical) can also inhibit your sexuality. A reduction or loss of oestrogen, testosterone and progesterone can mean that your sex drive reduces and vaginal dryness may make penetration painful. The surgery may also alter the shape of the vagina, especially if the cervix is removed, as this means it is shortened and/or tightened; and finally any scar tissue which forms can be painful if it is rubbed by the end of a penis. But there is some research that suggests, some of this can be simply down to a 'use it or lose it' effect, as it is becoming evident that normally sexually active women may avoid the worst drying changes to the vagina after menopause which are normally caused by a decline in oestrogen.

If you do have problems with physical changes, there may be no easy solutions. Your gynaecologist may brush them off, suggesting that sex at your age isn't something to worry about (believe me, it does happen) or say that artificial hormones or lubricating jellies will compensate. But, while they can be helpful, they are no substitute for the real thing, they may restore wetness to the vagina, but they don't do anything for a lack of arousal that would have stimulated the vaginal secretions in the first place.

You could also try hormone replacement therapy (ERT) as oestrogen restores vaginal tone and lubrication, progesterone may decrease depression (thereby increasing sexual interest), and testosterone increases your libido. A water based lubricant, such as KY Jelly, can provide artificial moisture in the vagina that will decrease painful penetration. While this doesn't substitute for natural arousal, by preventing pain it may stimulate your body's own natural processes, promoting relaxation and enjoyment.

If you are having problems with sex after hysterectomy do talk to your husband or partner as well, after all they aren't mind readers and many will probably welcome the opportunity to find out what is causing your change in response. When they are aware of the issues then they could become your biggest ally in finding a way through the minefield that will suit both of you.

But, what if you don't want to take HRT though? There are a number of supplements, herbs and dietary changes that could be beneficial. Discussing them all though, is really outside the scope of this book, but I have found Cathy Taylor's ebook, 'How to Conquer Menopause' (*www.tinyurl.com/fgwxt*), just about the best read of all. It is incredibly helpful, full of information and very supportive about every aspect of the menopause.

Sexuality

Let's face it though, our brains are the major sexual organ in our body, and how we feel about sex will profoundly affect our experience of it. Sex is very much about the physical, whilst sexuality is about our feelings and emotions. Getting our sexuality back on track can be quite a journey for some of us, and one that is often not experienced lightly.

Over the years, I have heard many stories from women that have contacted The Hysterectomy Association. I have also heard them from their husbands and partners and a common theme that emerges from those who are experiencing a problem is 'what's the point if I can't make babies?' Finding an alternative reason to enjoy sex is crucial to having a stimulating and ongoing relationship with our partners.

This attitude to sex is very much driven by how we were brought up to think about sex, whether it was in a positive or negative way can be very powerful drivers. The following things can all impact on how you view your sexuality after a hysterectomy:-

❖ Your parent's attitude to sex and displays of affection can be very influential. You may have been taught that sex is dirty and you shouldn't be doing 'it', or that hugging and kissing, especially in front of other people, is unwelcome. Alternatively you may have been brought up to be open in showing your affections and feelings and given positive messages about having loving sexual relationships.

❖ Cultural attitudes may suggest a woman's place is to be at home bringing up children. Your fertility can be seen as an asset to be taken with you to your husband's family, and so not being able to have children could damage your reputation as a *'good'* wife.

❖ Religious expectations of virginity and purity before marriage that you have had instilled into you could make you feel that your gynaecological problems are a 'punishment' for some wrong doing you have done in the past.

Over the years, and several husbands down the road, I have done a lot of work on my attitude to sex, and my own sexuality. I believe some of my problems may have stemmed from events in my childhood as I was badly affected by my brother's death when I was 10 years old and there is also a very strong possibility that my sister and I were sexually abused by a friend of the family at around the same time. Interestingly, there is a lot of research that is showing a strong link between undiagnosed pelvic pain and early sexual or physical abuse.

Until relatively recently I've never really had a successful sex life and I often wonder if those early experiences were at the root of some my problems, both sexual and physical. Slowly, over the years it has dawned on me that my sex life had been characterised by power plays – "if you do this for me, I'll do that for you". It had never really been about the joining together of two people in a common expression of their love, affection and regard for each other. In fact love never really came into it and if any ex-husbands or boyfriends are reading this, then I truly apologise for any trauma I may have caused you!

Although I never actually had penetration until I was 18, I did do almost everything else you could possibly do; and part of me 'learnt' that this was one way of creating relationships. As I got older, I realised it isn't particularly satisfying to be so bound up in power struggles, and finally with my husband John, I am finding a peace and contentment in our sex life that I have never had before – it has truly become a time that we share our love for each other. My sexuality has been awakened and it is no longer about just the physical, I can now say my mind is involved as well.

What about your own sexuality?

I'd like you to think a little about your own attitudes to sex and your sexuality. You might like to write or draw about how you feel. You might also like to think about how you believe your partner feels about you after your hysterectomy. If you are worried by his reaction to you, have you sat down and talked about it?

It might be helpful to try and answer the following questions:

1. What do you remember of your parent's attitude to affection and love? Were you openly demonstrative as a family or did it all go on 'behind closed doors'?
2. What do you know of your partners family attitudes to sex (quite often we pick partners – quite unconsciously – who have the same/similar backgrounds to ourselves)

3. Was your attitude to sex coloured by any early sexual encounters, particularly your first love? Have you ever explored how you were affected by them?

4. Has sex ever been used as a bargaining tool in your relationships?

5. Is sex just for one thing? – making babies or fulfilling marital obligations for instance

6. Have you ever been abused, sexually or physically? This might seem like an odd question to ask, but research is showing that women who have been abused do seem to suffer far more unexplained pelvic pain than those that haven't.

If any of these questions brings up issues for you, it might be helpful to talk them through with your partner (if you feel you can), a friend who can just listen without trying to offer advice or confidentially with a counsellor.

If you do have a past history of sexual or physical abuse that impacts on your relationship, I would suggest you to talk to either your GP or a counsellor, especially if you feel that it may be affecting your health, your sexuality or your recovery after hysterectomy. Appropriate counselling could provide the support and guidance that you need to help with any chronic pain you have, your emotional state and your recovery.

The End of My Story

And so to the end of my own story; after I had my hysterectomy, I divorced my then husband, met a lovely new man (John) and went back to University to take a Masters degree in Information Science. Part of my studies required me to do a thesis, and as I was interested in health information for patients I decided to draw on my own experience of having a hysterectomy. I looked at the part information plays in the experience of surgery, and the results shocked me.

The research showed that when a woman is given information, any amount, she had a much better experience of surgery than those who had not been given any at all. It seems that being given information by a medical professional is intimately bound up in the perception of levels of care we believe we have had. I know, it's obvious when you think about it but I realised how little I had known before my own operation and I sometimes wonder if my own decisions might have been different if I had known then, what I know now. The Hysterectomy Association was born as a direct result of doing that research, and each and every day I get more women contacting me who tell me the same thing, they don't have enough information – it appears that nothing has changed since the mid 1990's, and this is a worldwide phenomenon, not just limited to the

NHS and the UK. My mission in life, as I see it, is to provide women with enough impartial information and support so that they feel able to make an informed choice about what they need both physically and emotionally.

I have spent many years since my hysterectomy looking for the answers to explain my own experience and I finally feel as if I am getting there. It has often been a hard road to travel, but in many ways I am so glad I did – because it has changed me profoundly. I am not the same woman I was when I had my surgery, I know so much more than I did, I am more self aware, I am more assured and confident, I enjoy my sexuality and my femininity in ways I never felt allowed to before, and I have a life purpose. I wish the same for you!

With love, light and laughter

Linda x

Helping Yourself

So what can you do to help yourself if you do experience any of the problems that have been talked about in this book?

Initially it could be beneficial to ask "how do I think I may feel after I have had my hysterectomy?" You might recognise that you won't feel anything, you feel ready for the surgery and will be glad to get on with your life; however, you may realise that your womb is something that defines the 'real you' and that you will feel some grief if it is lost.

If you find after asking the question, you realise how much you are defined by your womb then investigating any possible alternatives to surgery, if they are appropriate/available for your condition, might be wise. If you aren't able to use any alternatives and a hysterectomy is really your only option then being really well informed about every aspect of the surgery, so that you know exactly what to expect would be advisable.

If you have feel you have made a well thought out, informed decision, and have allowed both yourself and your family enough time and resources to prepare for your hysterectomy, AND you feel that having the operation is the best choice in your situation, you will significantly minimise any possible emotional turmoil you might experience.

What if you have already had your hysterectomy?

If the reason for your emotional discomfort is purely physical or you are beginning to experience menopausal symptoms, and there isn't any underlying, deep-seated cause such as grief, then HRT may well help. It is important to remember though, that articles which might suggest that using HRT makes everything in your body "exactly as it was before" are misleading. This is because we don't know everything there is to know about the hormones that the ovaries produce, nor the complex processes their interaction causes.

Most HRT for those of us that have had a hysterectomy is oestrogen based, but if you are having problems with your libido then it might be worth asking about testosterone supplements as it helps to regulate sex drive, levels of energy and mood.

What if you don't want to use HRT?

If you prefer not to take HRT for any reason, then changing your diet, using supplements and herbs may be more acceptable to you, and may provide the physical support your body needs. Many reasons are given for not taking HRT; they include things like fear of breast cancer, unwelcome side effects or even a simple wish not to put extra chemicals in to our body.

Alternatively, many women have felt that natural progesterone creams are very beneficial to them; they are believed to help with symptoms such as loss of libido, depression (hormonal), hot flushes, night sweats and sleep disturbances. Recently published research is now suggesting that progesterone based contraceptives might be more beneficial, and have less risk attached, than the older combined pill. The same may well be found to be true of progesterone to manage the menopause.

Unfortunately you cannot be prescribed natural progesterone, but you can get it over the internet.

Alternatively, you could get one of the following books, which are all incredibly informative about what you can do with natural alternatives to HRT, such as herbs, supplements and diet.

- What Your Doctor May Not Tell You About Menopause: The Breakthrough Book on Natural Progesterone (*www.tinyurl.com/fdamx*)
- New Natural Alternatives To HRT (*www.tinyurl.com/pgya8*)
- The Premature Menopause Book (*www.tinyurl.com/roqmp*)

The most common natural approach is to look at supplementing your diet or changing it in some way so that it also incorporates naturally occurring hormones called phyto-oestrogens. These powerful and natural substances can be found in all sorts of food including Soya and linseed. As well as phyto-oestrogens a number of herbs are also said to be very helpful, such as Black Cohosh, which the North American Indians have used for generations to relieve menopausal symptoms.

Ten tips to supercharge your sex life

1. Talk about it with your partner – tell them what you like and why. Then ask your partner, things could have changed for them as well since you last discussed it!
2. Avoid having penetration for a while (particularly while healing), just stroking and touching can be very arousing.
3. Explore your fantasies with each other, talk about how you could surprise each other.
4. Do something different. Pinch his bottom, wink suggestively over the canapés at your neighbours Christmas party, do it in the hallway, on the stairs, in the car – in a quiet country lane, in the local woods or even book a hotel for the night.
5. Don't ignore the urge – your sex drive is like a muscle, it needs to be exercised
6. Don't put pressure on yourselves to perform – your sex life is unique, just like everything else about you. Contrary to the popular press the majority of the country are NOT doing it four times a week, there is no 'average'.
7. Try watching a sexy film together, you'll be surprised at just how much effect it can have on a woman
8. Arrange to get rid of the children, or the in-laws for the night and enjoy a bit of romance for change
9. Release your inner teenager – and laugh when you remember what your mother would have said
10. Give each other a massage with oils specially selected to arouse the senses.

What if my emotions are more deep-seated?

The purpose of this book has not been to frighten you, because the truth is that the majority of women will not suffer much in the way of emotional trauma. However, by knowing that there might be such an outcome to your surgery means you can prepare for it - and in that preparation lies strength. It is also important to remember at all times, that there is no right way to experience a hysterectomy; there is only your way. You are unique and what you feel is right for you, so please don't let anyone else tell you otherwise.

If you are experiencing anxiety, stress, grief, guilt, depression or even post traumatic stress, then it can be helpful talking to a counsellor. However, it is worth remembering that a simple acknowledgment of your feelings can be very powerful, and in 30% of cases depression will lift in its own time without any intervention at all. Go with it, if you feel like crying, then cry; if you feel like singing, sing. Express yourself in all the wonderful ways, only you know you can – and in that expression is healing, in fact self expression is one of the most powerful forms of healing we can ever know. The problems will come if you try to ignore or bury your emotions, this can lead to a deeper crisis in the long term and may mean you never fully recover your health.

By using the journaling part of this book, you can provide yourself with the acknowledgement you need. You need not share it with anyone else, but by being honest with yourself, you open the door to moving on in your life, as well as being able to cope with your distress more easily.

The Hysterectomy Association also offers counselling for women – and in some cases their partners – who are finding their hysterectomy overwhelming. You can contact us by email at *info@hysterectomy-association.org.uk* to make an appointment for an initial exploratory session. You can find out more about our counselling services on our website at *www.hysterectomy-association.org.uk/counsell/counsell.php*.

For those of you who are not so local to Dorset, we also offer online coaching. You can find out more about what coaching is and how it may help you from the website at *www.hysterectomy-association.org.uk/counsell/coaching.php*. Finally, I am creating a two day workshop called 'Losing the woman within'; more details will be posted on our website as soon as they are available.

Your Story

We would love to hear your story as well, and we may like to use it in later editions of this book and other publications if you would be happy for us to do so. Of course we will respect your privacy and keep anything you send anonymous unless you tell us otherwise.

How to Use Your Journal Pages

The journal pages are made up of both lined and unlined pages, there is one of each type for you to use and you can simply photocopy any extra sheets as you need them.

You will notice that there are a number of symbols at the bottom of each page, they could be a useful visual reminder of how you feel on any given day and I use the printed meanings for each one – you may like to write in alternative meanings that are more relevant for you.

☺	I feel happy	
☺	I feel neutral	
☹	I am feel sad	
✎	I'm OK	
✎	I'm not OK	
☠	I feel very ill	
✿	I feel mellow	
●	I am ready to explode	
♩	I just want peace	
☯	I'm OK, You're OK	
✌	Victory	
♪	I'm listening to my body	
?	I have so many questions	
✿	I'm putting on a brave face	

🔓	I think I've found the key	
𓅃	I am at peace	
🔌	I need urgent medical attention	
❤	I'm all loved up	

I have also included a scaling diary on each page, those of you that have read 101 Handy Hints for a Happy Hysterectomy will be familiar with the scaling diary concept, but for those that aren't I'll give a short explanation.

Mark on the diary where you are each day (even two or three times a day if you need to), it can help you to identify patterns in your physical and emotional states and can also help you to chart your progress, which at times can seem very slow. I have left a couple of blank scales so that you can measure progress in other areas as well if you would like to.

(1 is the worst you've had or done and 10 is the best you've had or done)

⊕ Pain	1	2	3	4	5	6	7	8	9	10
⊕ Sleeping	1	2	3	4	5	6	7	8	9	10
⊕ Mood	1	2	3	4	5	6	7	8	9	10
⊕ Tiredness	1	2	3	4	5	6	7	8	9	10
⊕ Walking/exercise	1	2	3	4	5	6	7	8	9	10
⊕ Sadness	1	2	3	4	5	6	7	8	9	10
⊕ Stress and Anxiety	1	2	3	4	5	6	7	8	9	10
	1	2	3	4	5	6	7	8	9	10
	1	2	3	4	5	6	7	8	9	10

Date

☺ ☺ ☹ 👍 👎 ☠ ✿ 💣 🏳 ☯ ✌ 👂 ? 🗡 🎭 🔓 🕊 🚑 ❤

_____

_____

_____

_____

_____

_____

_____

_____

_____

_____

_____

_____

_____

_____

_____

_____

_____

(1 is the worst you've had or done and 10 is the best you've had or done)

⊕ Pain	1	2	3	4	5	6	7	8	9	10
⊕ Sleeping	1	2	3	4	5	6	7	8	9	10
⊕ Mood	1	2	3	4	5	6	7	8	9	10
⊕ Tiredness	1	2	3	4	5	6	7	8	9	10
⊕ Walking/exercise	1	2	3	4	5	6	7	8	9	10
⊕ Sadness	1	2	3	4	5	6	7	8	9	10
⊕ Stress and Anxiety	1	2	3	4	5	6	7	8	9	10
	1	2	3	4	5	6	7	8	9	10
	1	2	3	4	5	6	7	8	9	10

Date
_____

☺ ☻ ☹ 👍 👎 ☠ ❀ 💣 ⚐ ☯ ✌ ✏ ? ✿ 🎭 🔓 🕊 📷 ❤

(1 is the worst you've had or done and 10 is the best you've had or done)

❋ Pain	1	2	3	4	5	6	7	8	9	10
❋ Sleeping	1	2	3	4	5	6	7	8	9	10
❋ Mood	1	2	3	4	5	6	7	8	9	10
❋ Tiredness	1	2	3	4	5	6	7	8	9	10
❋ Walking/exercise	1	2	3	4	5	6	7	8	9	10
❋ Sadness	1	2	3	4	5	6	7	8	9	10
❋ Stress and Anxiety	1	2	3	4	5	6	7	8	9	10
	1	2	3	4	5	6	7	8	9	10
	1	2	3	4	5	6	7	8	9	10

Date

☺ ☻ ☹ 👍 👎 ☠ ✿ 💣 🏳 ☯ ✌ 👂 ? 🗡 🎭 🔓 🕊 🚑 ♥

_____

_____

_____

_____

_____

_____

_____

_____

_____

_____

_____

_____

_____

_____

_____

_____

_____

_____

(1 is the worst you've had or done and 10 is the best you've had or done)

⊛ Pain	1	2	3	4	5	6	7	8	9	10
⊛ Sleeping	1	2	3	4	5	6	7	8	9	10
⊛ Mood	1	2	3	4	5	6	7	8	9	10
⊛ Tiredness	1	2	3	4	5	6	7	8	9	10
⊛ Walking/exercise	1	2	3	4	5	6	7	8	9	10
⊛ Sadness	1	2	3	4	5	6	7	8	9	10
⊛ Stress and Anxiety	1	2	3	4	5	6	7	8	9	10
	1	2	3	4	5	6	7	8	9	10
	1	2	3	4	5	6	7	8	9	10

Date

☺ ☺ ☹ 👍 ✌ ☠ ❀ 💣 🏳 ☯ ✌ 👂 ❓ 🗡 🦊 🔓 🕊 🚑 ♥

(1 is the worst you've had or done and 10 is the best you've had or done)

✹ Pain	1	2	3	4	5	6	7	8	9	10
✹ Sleeping	1	2	3	4	5	6	7	8	9	10
✹ Mood	1	2	3	4	5	6	7	8	9	10
✹ Tiredness	1	2	3	4	5	6	7	8	9	10
✹ Walking/exercise	1	2	3	4	5	6	7	8	9	10
✹ Sadness	1	2	3	4	5	6	7	8	9	10
✹ Stress and Anxiety	1	2	3	4	5	6	7	8	9	10
	1	2	3	4	5	6	7	8	9	10
	1	2	3	4	5	6	7	8	9	10

Date

☺ ☻ ☹ 👍 👎 ☠ ✿ 💣 🏳 ☯ ✌ 👂 ? 🗡 🎭 🔓 🕊 🚑 ♥

_____

_____

_____

_____

_____

_____

_____

_____

_____

_____

_____

_____

_____

_____

_____

_____

(1 is the worst you've had or done and 10 is the best you've had or done)

✿ Pain	1	2	3	4	5	6	7	8	9	10
✿ Sleeping	1	2	3	4	5	6	7	8	9	10
✿ Mood	1	2	3	4	5	6	7	8	9	10
✿ Tiredness	1	2	3	4	5	6	7	8	9	10
✿ Walking/exercise	1	2	3	4	5	6	7	8	9	10
✿ Sadness	1	2	3	4	5	6	7	8	9	10
✿ Stress and Anxiety	1	2	3	4	5	6	7	8	9	10
	1	2	3	4	5	6	7	8	9	10
	1	2	3	4	5	6	7	8	9	10

Date

☺ ☻ ☹ 👍 👎 ☠ ❀ 💣 🏳 ◑ ✌ 👂 ? 🔪 🎲 🔓 🕊 🚑 ♥

(1 is the worst you've had or done and 10 is the best you've had or done)

	1	2	3	4	5	6	7	8	9	10
❀ Pain	1	2	3	4	5	6	7	8	9	10
❀ Sleeping	1	2	3	4	5	6	7	8	9	10
❀ Mood	1	2	3	4	5	6	7	8	9	10
❀ Tiredness	1	2	3	4	5	6	7	8	9	10
❀ Walking/exercise	1	2	3	4	5	6	7	8	9	10
❀ Sadness	1	2	3	4	5	6	7	8	9	10
❀ Stress and Anxiety	1	2	3	4	5	6	7	8	9	10
	1	2	3	4	5	6	7	8	9	10
	1	2	3	4	5	6	7	8	9	10

Date

☺ ☺ ☺ 👍 👎 ☠ ✿ 💣 🏳 ☯ ✌ 👂 ❓ 🗡 🎭 🔓 🕊 🚑 ♥

_____

_____

_____

_____

_____

_____

_____

_____

_____

_____

_____

_____

_____

_____

_____

_____

(1 is the worst you've had or done and 10 is the best you've had or done)

✿ Pain	1	2	3	4	5	6	7	8	9	10
✿ Sleeping	1	2	3	4	5	6	7	8	9	10
✿ Mood	1	2	3	4	5	6	7	8	9	10
✿ Tiredness	1	2	3	4	5	6	7	8	9	10
✿ Walking/exercise	1	2	3	4	5	6	7	8	9	10
✿ Sadness	1	2	3	4	5	6	7	8	9	10
✿ Stress and Anxiety	1	2	3	4	5	6	7	8	9	10
	1	2	3	4	5	6	7	8	9	10
	1	2	3	4	5	6	7	8	9	10

Date

_____

☺ ☻ ☹ 👍 👎 ☠ ❀ 💣 🏳 🌀 ✌ 👂 ? 🗡 🎴 🔓 🕊 🚑 ❤

(1 is the worst you've had or done and 10 is the best you've had or done)

❀ Pain	1	2	3	4	5	6	7	8	9	10
❀ Sleeping	1	2	3	4	5	6	7	8	9	10
❀ Mood	1	2	3	4	5	6	7	8	9	10
❀ Tiredness	1	2	3	4	5	6	7	8	9	10
❀ Walking/exercise	1	2	3	4	5	6	7	8	9	10
❀ Sadness	1	2	3	4	5	6	7	8	9	10
❀ Stress and Anxiety	1	2	3	4	5	6	7	8	9	10
	1	2	3	4	5	6	7	8	9	10
	1	2	3	4	5	6	7	8	9	10

Date

_____

☺ ☺ ☺ 👍 👎 ☠ ✿ 💣 🏳 ☯ ✌ 👂 **?** 🗡 🎭 🔓 🕊 🚑 ♥

_____
_____
_____
_____
_____
_____
_____
_____
_____
_____
_____
_____
_____
_____
_____
_____
_____
_____

(1 is the worst you've had or done and 10 is the best you've had or done)

✾ Pain	1	2	3	4	5	6	7	8	9	10
✾ Sleeping	1	2	3	4	5	6	7	8	9	10
✾ Mood	1	2	3	4	5	6	7	8	9	10
✾ Tiredness	1	2	3	4	5	6	7	8	9	10
✾ Walking/exercise	1	2	3	4	5	6	7	8	9	10
✾ Sadness	1	2	3	4	5	6	7	8	9	10
✾ Stress and Anxiety	1	2	3	4	5	6	7	8	9	10
	1	2	3	4	5	6	7	8	9	10
	1	2	3	4	5	6	7	8	9	10

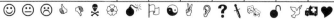

☺ ☺ ☺ 👍 👎 ☠ ✿ 💣 🏳 ☯ ✌ 👂 **?** 🗡 🎭 🔓 🕊 🚑 ♥

Date

_____

(1 is the worst you've had or done and 10 is the best you've had or done)

⊕ Pain	1	2	3	4	5	6	7	8	9	10
⊕ Sleeping	1	2	3	4	5	6	7	8	9	10
⊕ Mood	1	2	3	4	5	6	7	8	9	10
⊕ Tiredness	1	2	3	4	5	6	7	8	9	10
⊕ Walking/exercise	1	2	3	4	5	6	7	8	9	10
⊕ Sadness	1	2	3	4	5	6	7	8	9	10
⊕ Stress and Anxiety	1	2	3	4	5	6	7	8	9	10
	1	2	3	4	5	6	7	8	9	10
	1	2	3	4	5	6	7	8	9	10

Date

_____

☺ ☺ ☺ 👍 👎 ☠ ❀ 💣 🏳 ☯ ✌ 👂 ? 🗡 🎭 🔓 🕊 🚑 ♥

_____
_____
_____
_____
_____
_____
_____
_____
_____
_____
_____
_____
_____
_____
_____
_____

(1 is the worst you've had or done and 10 is the best you've had or done)

❀ Pain	1	2	3	4	5	6	7	8	9	10
❀ Sleeping	1	2	3	4	5	6	7	8	9	10
❀ Mood	1	2	3	4	5	6	7	8	9	10
❀ Tiredness	1	2	3	4	5	6	7	8	9	10
❀ Walking/exercise	1	2	3	4	5	6	7	8	9	10
❀ Sadness	1	2	3	4	5	6	7	8	9	10
❀ Stress and Anxiety	1	2	3	4	5	6	7	8	9	10
	1	2	3	4	5	6	7	8	9	10
	1	2	3	4	5	6	7	8	9	10

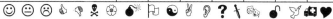
☺ ☺ ☺ 👍 👎 ☠ ❀ 💣 🏳 ☯ ✌ 👂 ? 🗡 🎭 🔓 🕊 🚑 ♥

Date

(1 is the worst you've had or done and 10 is the best you've had or done)

⊛ Pain	1	2	3	4	5	6	7	8	9	10
⊛ Sleeping	1	2	3	4	5	6	7	8	9	10
⊛ Mood	1	2	3	4	5	6	7	8	9	10
⊛ Tiredness	1	2	3	4	5	6	7	8	9	10
⊛ Walking/exercise	1	2	3	4	5	6	7	8	9	10
⊛ Sadness	1	2	3	4	5	6	7	8	9	10
⊛ Stress and Anxiety	1	2	3	4	5	6	7	8	9	10
	1	2	3	4	5	6	7	8	9	10
	1	2	3	4	5	6	7	8	9	10

Date

☺ ☺ ☹ 👍 👎 ☠ ❀ 💣 🏳 ☯ ✌ 👂 ? 🗡 🎭 🔓 🕊 🚑 ♥

_____

_____

_____

_____

_____

_____

_____

_____

_____

_____

_____

_____

_____

_____

_____

_____

(1 is the worst you've had or done and 10 is the best you've had or done)

❀ Pain	1	2	3	4	5	6	7	8	9	10
❀ Sleeping	1	2	3	4	5	6	7	8	9	10
❀ Mood	1	2	3	4	5	6	7	8	9	10
❀ Tiredness	1	2	3	4	5	6	7	8	9	10
❀ Walking/exercise	1	2	3	4	5	6	7	8	9	10
❀ Sadness	1	2	3	4	5	6	7	8	9	10
❀ Stress and Anxiety	1	2	3	4	5	6	7	8	9	10
	1	2	3	4	5	6	7	8	9	10
	1	2	3	4	5	6	7	8	9	10

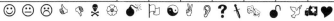

☺ ☺ ☹ 👍 👎 ☠ ❀ 💣 🏳 ☯ ✌ 👂 ? 🗡 🎭 🔓 🕊 🚑 ♥

Date

_____

(1 is the worst you've had or done and 10 is the best you've had or done)

⊛ Pain	1	2	3	4	5	6	7	8	9	10
⊛ Sleeping	1	2	3	4	5	6	7	8	9	10
⊛ Mood	1	2	3	4	5	6	7	8	9	10
⊛ Tiredness	1	2	3	4	5	6	7	8	9	10
⊛ Walking/exercise	1	2	3	4	5	6	7	8	9	10
⊛ Sadness	1	2	3	4	5	6	7	8	9	10
⊛ Stress and Anxiety	1	2	3	4	5	6	7	8	9	10
	1	2	3	4	5	6	7	8	9	10
	1	2	3	4	5	6	7	8	9	10

Date

☺ ☻ ☹ 👍 👎 ☠ ✿ 💣 🚩 ☯ ✌ 👂 ? 🗡 🎭 🔒 🕊 🚑 ♥

_____

_____

_____

_____

_____

_____

_____

_____

_____

_____

_____

_____

_____

_____

_____

(1 is the worst you've had or done and 10 is the best you've had or done)

⊛ Pain	1	2	3	4	5	6	7	8	9	10
⊛ Sleeping	1	2	3	4	5	6	7	8	9	10
⊛ Mood	1	2	3	4	5	6	7	8	9	10
⊛ Tiredness	1	2	3	4	5	6	7	8	9	10
⊛ Walking/exercise	1	2	3	4	5	6	7	8	9	10
⊛ Sadness	1	2	3	4	5	6	7	8	9	10
⊛ Stress and Anxiety	1	2	3	4	5	6	7	8	9	10
	1	2	3	4	5	6	7	8	9	10
	1	2	3	4	5	6	7	8	9	10

Working On Your Fear and Anxiety

MY FEAR IS?

I WILL TALK TO THE FOLLOWING PEOPLE ABOUT IT

THEIR ANSWER WAS ...

Working On Your Fear and Anxiety

MY FEAR IS?

I WILL TALK TO THE FOLLOWING PEOPLE ABOUT IT

THEIR ANSWER WAS ...

Resources

Hysterectomy

The Hysterectomy Association, 0871 7811141
www.hysterectomy-association.org.uk

Menopause

The British Menopause Society, 01628 890199
http://www.the-bms.org/

The Daisy Network
http://www.daisynetwork.org.uk/

North American Menopause Society, 440/442-7550
http://www.menopause.org/default.htm

Australasian Menopause Society, 61 3 6391 3122
http://www.menopause.org.au/

Hormone Replacement Therapy

Women's Health Initiative, 1 800 994 9662
http://www.4woman.gov/menopause/news.htm

Infertility

Fertility Society Australia, (03) 9645 6359
http://www.fsa.au.com/

Infertility Network UK
http://www.infertilitynetworkuk.com/

Resolve, 301-652-8585
http://www.resolve.org/site/PageServer

Abortion

Marie Stopes International, 0845 300 80 90

http://www.abortion-help.co.uk/

National **Abortion** and Reproductive Rights Action League, 202.973.3000
http://www.naral.org/

Marie Stopes International Australia, 1800 003 707
http://www.mariestopes.com.au/

Bibliography

Pandey SK, Hart JJ, Tiwary S; *Women's Health and the Internet: Understanding Emerging Trends and Implications;* Soc Sci Med. 2003;56:179-191

A Prescription for a New View of Women's Positive Sexual Health
 - (http://www.medscape.com/viewarticle/457785?src=search)

Karen M. Hicks, PhD, *The "New View" Approach to Women's Sexual Problems CME/CE*
 - (http://health.yahoo.com/ency/healthwise/tv1976)

The Hysterectomy Book - (http://www.shb.ie/content611260702_1.cfm)

Clark, J. *Hysterectomy and the alternatives*; London 2000

Maas CP; Kenter GG; Trimbos JB; Deruiter MC; *Anatomical basis for nerve-sparing radical hysterectomy: immunohistochemical study of the pelvic autonomic nerves.* Acta Obstet Gynecol Scand. 2005; 84(9):868-74 (ISSN: 0001-6349)

Gütl P; Greimel ER; Roth R; Winter R; *Women's sexual behavior, body image and satisfaction with surgical outcomes after hysterectomy: a comparison of vaginal and abdominal surgery.* J Psychosom Obstet Gynaecol. 2002; 23(1):51-9 (ISSN: 0167-482X)

Maas CP; ter Kuile MM; Laan E; Tuijnman CC; Weijenborg PT; Trimbos JB; Kenter GG; *Objective assessment of sexual arousal in women with a history of hysterectomy.* BJOG. 2004; 111(5):456-62 (ISSN: 1470-0328)

Lowenstein L; Yarnitsky D; Gruenwald I; Deutsch M; Sprecher E; Gedalia U; Vardi Y; *Does hysterectomy affect genital sensation?* Eur J Obstet Gynecol Reprod Biol. 2005; 119(2):242-5 (ISSN: 0301-2115)

DeAngelo, D. *Sudden Menopause*; Dublin, 2002

Greer, G. *The Whole Woman*; London, 1999

Parker, W. H. *A Gynaecologists Second Opinion*; Middlesex 1996

Goldfarb, H. A. & Greif, J. *The No Hysterectomy Option, your body your choice*; Canada, 1997

Mackinger HF; Graf AH; Keck E; Tempfer C; Kainz C, *Differences in the psychological status of hysterectomy and non-hysterectomy women.* Wien Klin Wochenschr. 2001; 113(23-24):954-9 (ISSN: 0043-5325)

Aziz A; Bergquist C; Brännström M; Nordholm L; Silfverstolpe; *Differences in aspects of personality and sexuality between perimenopausal women making different choices regarding prophylactic oophorectomy at elective hysterectomy.* Acta Obstet Gynecol Scand. 2005; 84(9):854-9 (ISSN: 0001-6349)

Laurie Barclay, MD, CME Author: Charles Vega, MD, FAAFP; *ACOG Issues New Guidelines for Chronic Pelvic Pain* CME

Poleshuck EL; Dworkin RH; Howard FM; Foster DC; Shields CG; Giles DE; Tu X; *Contributions of physical and sexual abuse to women's experiences with chronic pelvic pain.* J Reprod Med. 2005; 50(2):91-100 (ISSN: 0024-7758)

Thomas E; Moss-Morris R; Faquhar C, *Coping with emotions and abuse history in women with chronic pelvic pain.* J Psychosom Res. 2006; 60(1):109-12 (ISSN: 0022-3999)

Hahn L; *Chronic pelvic pain in women. A condition difficult to diagnose--more than 70 different diagnoses can be considered.* Lakartidningen. 2001; 98(15):1780-5 (ISSN: 0023-7205)

Nijenhuis ER; van Dyck R; ter Kuile MM; Mourits MJ; Spinhoven P; van der Hart O, *Evidence for associations among somatoform dissociation, psychological dissociation and reported trauma in patients with chronic pelvic pain.* J Psychosom Obstet Gynaecol. 2003; 24(2):87-98 (ISSN: 0167-482X)

Hilden M; Schei B; Swahnberg K; Halmesmäki E; Langhoff-Roos J; Offerdal K; Pikarinen U; Sidenius K; Steingrimsdottir T; Stoum-Hinsverk H; Wijma B; *A history of sexual abuse and health: a Nordic multicentre study.* BJOG. 2004; 111(10):1121-7 (ISSN: 1470-0328)

Lampe A; Doering S; Rumpold G; Sölder E; Krismer M; Kantner-Rumplmair W; Schubert C; Söllner W; *Chronic pain syndromes and their relation to childhood abuse and stressful life events.* J Psychosom Res. 2003; 54(4):361-7 (ISSN: 0022-3999)

Poleshuck EL; Dworkin RH; Howard FM; Foster DC; Shields CG; Giles DE; Tu X; *Contributions of physical and sexual abuse to women's experiences with chronic pelvic pain.* J Reprod Med. 2005; 50(2):91-100 (ISSN: 0024-7758)

Made in the USA
Middletown, DE
26 May 2017